Losing Weight with Jogging

How beginners can quickly burn fat

From equipment to correct nutrition

Andreas Graf

Published by

JoelNoah S.A.

info@joelnoah.com

Author: Andreas Graf

Losing Weight with Jogging

How beginners can quickly burn fat

From equipment to correct nutrition

Copyright 2013 by JoelNoah S.A.

ISBN-13: 978-1493762804

ISBN-10: 149376280X

Edition License Notes

Table of Contents

Introduction

Nowadays, many people carry around "a couple of extra pounds". That's reason enough to finally start with a type of sport which will gradually and gently reduce their weight.

Jogging has many benefits which not only address slender and athletic people, but also help beginners in running, with weight problems, to feel better bodily and to have an increased mobility.

However, there are some important criteria which must be observed. Training through running is supposed to be fun, and in the long term, it should motivate even joggers with overweight to move regularly. Whoever puts the advice into practice, whatever his weight, will reap the benefits that result from a continuous running training, without negatively affecting joints, ligaments, or other parts of the musculoskeletal system.

Running shoes – innovative technologies for all requirements

Anybody who wants to do it can start running at any place or time. However, if you ever had to put up with the consequences of shoes that didn't fit perfectly, you know that wrong shoes will spoil the fun of walking or running.

People who are just getting started with the sport of running, and who don't find their way on the market, should get professional help in a specialized shop and have a lot of time available. Buying shoes is always a matter of trust, and especially running shoes must be appropriate for individual requirements.

Anybody who has overweight and wants to start a running training successfully must start slowly with the training program, and do so with optimal running shoes. Not just the body weight is important when selecting running shoes, but also the preferred distance profile and possible foot problems.

The most common position problems in the feet include the buckling foot, which bends inward when rolling the foot. For this problem, so-called stable running shoes, which include a special pronation support and provide stability to the foot without constricting it, are appropriate.

An optimal lacing is also important, if the person who runs wants to move freely. The foot must be fixed during running, without getting an unpleasant feeling due to a lacing that is too tight.

An excellent fit is ensured by the classic pulling system over the central part of the sole; each runner can decide for himself how tightly the running shoe should be on the foot.

The type of shoe laces is also important. Unlike triathletes, who require changing shoes quickly, runners should refrain from using round shoe laces, which can easily get untied while running.

How can a person, and especially a beginning runner, recognize a good shoe?

Basically, such a shoe should fulfill all the criteria which runners, including runners with overweight, require from a running shoe. Thus, for example, the size and weight of a runner affect the quality of absorption and stability elements, which have an enormous effect on the support and running comfort.

The heel and ball area of the feet are exposed to a great load for any runner, and have to be protected with a flexible outer sole. In a high-quality running shoe, this is characterized by a so-called flex notch, which separates both areas from the rest of the sole.

A running shoe's outer material should also have flexible quality traits. The foot should get enough freedom of movement from a supporting upper material to let it roll off on any ground, and yet be protected from irregularities such as stones and sticks.

It is often precisely people with some overweight who have problems with the balls of their feet. Stretchy and flexible insets are oriented towards the requirements of the balls of the feet, and also offer a high level of breathing activity. In addition, many running shoes have an inset from mesh material on their upper part; a coarse mesh allows the best air circulation, achieving a healthy environment for the feet.

You can also choose the weight of running shoes individually. However, this is only relevant for runners who want to participate in races at a high speed. For beginning runners and for long-distance runners, the weight of the shoes is rather irrelevant.

Competent advisors in professional shops assist and also take into account the clients desires. The ground for running, as well as the foot shape, individual problems and wrong positions as well as the runner's weight are taken into account, before the client makes his decision.

It is getting increasingly common for professional sports shops to offer treadmills and other technologies to find the individually appropriate model, in the best interest of the client. An analysis on a treadmill is an ideal way to find the appropriate running shoes, which combine stability and flexibility.

Ideally, training shoes should only be bought in the afternoon, since it is then that the feet have extended to their daily average, thus avoiding incorrect purchases of running shoes that are too tight. Bringing your own running socks also helps you choose the correct size, since the normal size of street shoes can usually not be applied to running shoes, which are normally one number bigger.

Clothing for running: Functionality is decisive

Whereas in the past sweaty runners ran around their tracks with cotton clothing, more recent developments have created sports fashion from innovative materials, which achieve a pleasant body environment.

A mixture of functionality and design leaves no desire unfulfilled, and even on cool days, thick and heavy running clothing belongs to the past. Modern fibers offer wind- and water repellant properties, provide breathability and ensure an ideal moisture exchange.

Sweat is carried out, without letting humidity get in. Special membranes achieve these important properties and persuade with an extremely light weight.

Running tights are comfortable pants made from elastic materials and having a cut that places them close to the body. They are also offered in large sizes, consist of breathable artificial fibers, can be washed in a washing machine without any problem and dry quickly. Jackets and running shirts also offer the same properties. Manufacturers have adapted to the desires of runners and offer a large variety, leaving no wish unfulfilled.

The runner decides whether he wants to use short or long sleeves. Models in which the sleeves can be taken off with a zipper are especially handy.

In any case, modern functional underwear should complement the sport clothing. Clothing without seams protects from pressure points, which makes it more comfortable to wear.

Having untarnished fun while running obviously also requires functional and high-quality running socks. They make a valuable complement for the individually fitting shoe, and should be part of any runner's basic equipment. Socks that don't fit well can cause painful friction and blisters, since just a small crease is enough to cause a disaster after just a few kilometers. High-quality running shoes take sweat to the outside even at high temperatures and high strain, without affecting how they fit. Skin-favorable mesh insets in the area of the central foot increase this effect and achieve additional stability, to continue providing the desired effect even after running several kilometers. If you want to protect yourself from chafing and blisters, you should use high-quality running socks.

Nowadays, people with overweight who want to protect their leg muscles can also use the benefits of compression socks. Developed in the past in the medical area for patients with circulatory problems, nowadays manufacturers of sport clothing also use them. Compression socks for running have a long shaft which consists of the same material from the ankle upwards, up to where the knee starts. This achieves a balanced pressure on the calve muscles.

As a result, not only are the arteries expanded to make it easier for them to transport blood, but oxygen transport to individual muscles is also assisted. Every runner should check individually whether wearing these compression socks makes it more pleasant to run, or whether a classic running sock is sufficient.

Medical examinations are a must for beginning runners

Any type of sports activity implies a certain amount of stress for the body. Especially people who are over 35 years old, and anybody who has problems with overweight, should not do without a physical examination for sports, when they want to start with some sort of sport. This special fitness for sport examination should be repeated once a year to preclude body problems.

The medical history as well as the current health status and special individual risk factors such as smoking, increased blood fat values and body weight are all considered in such an examination.

In cooperation with physicians, and considering any possible health risks, any patient can set up a running training program. The running speed and the extent of a training program can be determined based on the results of the physical examination; as a result, even recreational athletes with existing health problems can get the benefits of bodily activity.

Problems with the feet's musculoskeletal system are often solved with high-quality inlays, and even people with considerable overweight need not refrain from enjoying jogging. Ideally, people with a lot of overweight would first swim or ride bikes, and only start running after a while.

Warming up – an optimal start for any running program

Sport is favorable for health and it is supposed to be fun. However, it is important to prepare properly. An ample warming-up training should definitely be part of it, regardless of the distance you run.

Warming up prepares the muscles for running. The body should get to the ideal "operating temperature" of ca. 38.5 °C, to increase the circulation which is responsible for increased muscle tautness; this also has a positive influence on metabolism. This will reduce the risk of irritating ligaments and tendons and make the muscles more susceptible for cramps. A well-planned warming-up phase also prepares other parts of the body for physical activity. Thus, even the joints benefit from warming up, since the production of joint lubrication is stimulated, making the musculoskeletal system suppler, even in the case of people with overweight.

In addition, any runner can also use the warming up and stretching to prepare mentally for the running training. The main objective of the warming-up phase is to loosen the muscles, and this phase should adapt to the runner's requirements. Warming up should never be more tiring than the running training itself; rather, it should prepare you in a targeted and gentle way for the kilometers you will run.

Anybody who decides to train running ought to know that almost all muscle groups are stressed by this sport. Therefore it is sensible to get all muscle groups involved during the warm-up.

Runners like to use relaxed warm-up running. In a trot, especially the legs muscle groups are prepared. If you want to benefit from an effective running style, you should also include your torso.

Something that is easy to carry out even by people with overweight is marching on the spot during three minutes, complemented by running backwards slowly. Pushups and squats during three to four minutes as well as relaxing circular movements by the torso complement the warm-up phase.

To bring the body to the appropriate running temperature, runners should wear warm clothing, which are taken off during the running itself.

The running speed is subject to your personal capacity

The correct amount is essential! This principle is especially important for sport beginners, since it is not always easy to find a correct running speed when training.

Precisely people who are just getting started with running have a tendency to overestimate their own capacity. If beginning runners decide to train in groups, many of them have the risk of wanting to keep up with faster runners. However, it is important to make an objective self-assessment, if you want your body to continue feeling good after the training.

Only a runner who doesn't expose himself permanently to demands that are too high continues enjoying running in the future. If you get muscle soreness after training, this is a sure sign that your body has performed more than it can currently handle.

Especially beginning runners who have overweight should choose a realistic running speed, and anybody who has problems to find the correct speed would do well to use a heart rate monitor. This handy tool lets you find the speed that is appropriate for you individually, without overtaxing yourself.

Normally a heart rate monitor consists of straps with which the heart frequency can be measured. Safety-oriented runners who want to check their heart rate while running will find their appropriate individual long-term running speed.

Persistence sports such as swimming, riding bicycles and running can quickly overtax the body. The heart rate is a reliable parameter to measure the stress on the heart and the circulatory system. The so-called training pulse can be determined quickly by non-experts. The optimal value is 180 minus the age; 10 beats up or down can be included as tolerance.

Comfortable breast straps for runners transmit the data via radio waves to a special heart rate watch which the runner wears on his wrist. Modern devices are offered in different models, which may include a stop watch, an alarm, or even data storage.

People who want to play it safe will find their own rhythm by running regularly and at first slowly. If you want to participate in competitions, you can increase the running speed gradually, according to the training status.

It is not just the muscles which react to different running speeds, but also the metabolism. Especially people with overweight complain about a sluggish metabolism. If you decide to take up running, you can reactivate your metabolism by running at different speeds.

In the case of short distances, running at a high speed, the body uses carbohydrates to obtain energy. These are available as glycogen which can be used more efficiently than fat, even for high performance. If the running training continues for more than half an hour, the glycogen reserves are no longer able to satisfy the energy requirements. Rather, fat storage is used, which different runners have available in different quantities.

Basically, fat is an important energy provider, and a well-functioning metabolism isn't possible without fat. Thus, the overweight runner will benefit from running, as an appropriate way to lose fat. You'll find more about optimal nutrition in the chapter "**Lose weight healthily and quickly when jogging**".

The general rule is that fat loss is much higher in the case of a long-distance run at a moderate speed than running a short distance quickly. Every beginning runner must find his individually appropriate speed, according to the time spent running.

A balanced training, including one for overweight people, is based on simple but effective principles.

If you want to avoid the greatest running error, you should abstain from a high speed at the beginning of a training period. It makes more sense to run calmly during the first 15-20 minutes, and then carefully increase the speed.

It is not less effective to stop suddenly after the running. Instead, it is better for your health and circulation if you run the last few minutes to the goal at a slower speed.

The individual situation as well as experience with running determine the appropriate running speed, to let runners, including those that are overweight, feel well and regenerate quickly.

So-called slow-starts are quite popular. If at the beginning of a training session or a competition you go too quickly, you get exhausted quickly and will complain about muscle soreness for days. Even if an individual's circulatory system adapts quickly to a higher speed, other bodily systems usually take longer to do so.

If a beginning runner starts at peak performance, he will damage his health. International studies show that even running sessions of only ten minutes increase the body's capacity. At the same time the heart rate will improve long-term, and the person will start to quickly lose weight.

Sport scientists recommend anybody who aims for a ten-kilometer distance to run once a week in three sessions of 40 minutes each.

An individually appropriate training time requires sensitivity

You can observe it over and over again: Precisely beginning runners exaggerate in relation to the speed and time of a training session. However, nobody should overestimate his capacity; only a gradual increase of the effort will result in longer training distances, which can be run without negative effects on health.

A modern and healthy running training, including for athletes who have a few extra pounds, includes gradually increasing fitness. Anybody who carries out a training session too quickly and too intensively risks his health, and risks damage to his ligaments, tendons and articulations.

The desired goal of healthy running training is to gradually increase the body effort, to allow the body functions to adapt gradually to them. The body learns over time to take up more oxygen, and to adapt to the general stimuli, to thus positively affect the metabolism processes.

When having training sessions that are too long, beginners risk subjecting the body to too much effort, since it can no longer process the stimuli. In the worst case, an excessive training can even result in not gradually increasing the performance, but rather cause the runner great problems to withstand the effort. As a result, the beginning runner might not only stop enjoying the training, but also damage his health in the long term. Ultimately, an organism subjected to too much effort is more vulnerable to injuries and diseases. This not only affects older semesters and beginning runners with overweight, but also young people who overestimate their capabilities.

A person's physique as well as his weight affect the body's capacity. A healthy running training is successful if the general condition of the body is used as a measuring stick. Even beginners get great training results if at first they carry out a relaxed running training, which stimulates the burning of fat. The running speed and time can be increased gradually within three or four months.

A person who documents his training status can, as a beginner, also control his effort and relaxation phases. Basically, when running, anybody should pay attention to the body's signs, and adapt his training to that. Wrong movement sequences which cause an excessive effort or even injuries can be corrected. A straight posture and, initially, small running steps require a small effort. This can be used to gradually increase the duration of the running, and to stimulate the fat burning process.

Especially overweight people will find that an effective running training offers ideal conditions to reduce their body weight. A beginning runner who wants to do it correctly should also get familiar with directed power training. The emphasis here is on strengthening the muscles of the back of the lower and upper legs. Pushups and exercises for the back stretch muscles can also be carried out without any problems at home.

An efficient strengthening of leg muscles is also achieved when the runner does two or three runs a month in hilly terrain. Strong muscles not only prevent injuries to ligaments and tendons, they also improve the running economy.

Breathing: more than just getting air

Breathing is as important as having appropriate running shoes, running at the correct speed and individually adjusting the running time. Especially beginning runners often have to deal with wrong breathing, which quickly causes painful side stitches. However, there are simple tips which can help any runner breathe.

The effort during running training influences the breathing activity. Exhaling continuously and strongly forces you to inhale again, to provide the body with sufficient oxygen.

The classic belly breathing can be trained without problems, to make it work by itself when running. When inhaling, the abdominal wall is pressed outward, while when exhaling it is pulled in. A person who decides to breathe this way avoids breathing problems, even as an overweight beginning runner.

Normally for classic endurance running, breathing through the nose is sufficient. Only when the speed is increased will you start breathing through the mouth.

However, be careful in the cold season. Sensitive people risk getting a throat infection, since unlike when you breathe through the nose, the cold air is not warmed up when inhaling. In that case, runners should reduce their speed, to do their running with less air.

The correct posture – avoid back problems

If you believe that when running everything is just about legs and feet, get ready for a painful surprise. An incorrect posture when jogging can quickly cause back pain; therefore it is very important to pay attention to a correct posture.

Precisely beginning runners tend to pull up their shoulder area tensely and to keep their arms in a stiff position. Other runners swing their arms and make rowing movements, resulting in an ineffective running style and wasting energy.

Ideally, both arms should be slightly and loosely bent, and slightly move to the rhythm of the running movements. The pendulum movements should not go higher than the breast. An economical position of the arms also includes having the hands relaxed. Clenched and tense fists are harmful for a relaxed running style. The hands must be open and, if necessary, can also be slightly shaken around.

The backbone is also essential for relaxed running. The torso is bent slightly forwards, to avoid a hunchbacked posture or a hollow back. If the legs' movements correspond to arms that move in a relaxed way, you can avoid painful tensions in the back muscles even after a long training session.

Is the ground relevant?

Running is especially ideal for a healthy hearth-circulatory training; it stimulates the immune system and also liberates happiness hormones. But what about the ground?

With every step done when running, the leg accelerates the body and must cushion a considerable part of the body weight when landing. In the process, especially the knee, jumping and hip joints are strained with several times the normal body.

If a runner prefers concrete or asphalt streets, this ground doesn't yield, and the strain on joints and muscles increases. The result is often painful strains, when inexperienced runners prefer to run for longer distances on a hard ground.

According to insiders, an asphalt cover is also known as a "bone killer". However, many running trainers don't consider the risks that result from a hard ground to be that important.

The possibility of snapping over or slipping on asphalt is very small, and anybody who ever ran on the beach knows how easily you can get painful strains on a ground that yields.

Still, forest and meadow paths are considered ideal for having good training conditions, to go easy on joints and ligaments, especially for overweight runners. Besides, training on the forest floor also ensures that both the runner's coordination and his reflexes are trained well.

Special running techniques simplify training

In principle, anybody can run, but nowadays anybody who wants to be geared towards specific techniques will find three different variations, adapted to the runners' individual requirements and conditions: running with the front part, the middle part and the back part of the foot.

Running with the front part of the foot, also known as ball of the foot running, causes a great stress on the calves and the Achilles tendon. Only few runners manage to use this method for long distances, since the foot is placed on the floor above the ball of the big toe and the middle foot, up to the heel. This running technique is not very appropriate for beginners and should only be used once you are well trained.

Running with the middle part of the foot is less stressful; the tendons and joints are subjected to less stress, since the foot is placed on the floor above the heel.

Running with the back part of the foot is the most common way to run. Many running shoe manufacturers have adapted to this and optimize their models for the requirements that result from this running style. Here, the heel is placed on the ground in a steep angle, and then rolls off.

If as a beginning runner you don't want to get used to train a specific style, after a while you'll find your own style, adapted to your own body weight.

The running technique and the posture have an important role. If beginners develop a wrong running style, especially people with overweight have the risk of having problems in the area of their tendons, muscles and vertebra.

Running consists of two phases: support, and floating. While the foot is supported during the contact with the ground, the floating phase, among others, affects the length of the steps. This depends not only on the runner's size, but also on his body weight. A person who chooses a running temp that is not adapted to the body situation not only chooses an uneconomical running style, but also increases excessive strains.

Thus, you should take steps that are neither too long nor too short, but rather pay attention to a fluid and harmonic running style, according to the individual body situation.

Not much time, but still want to train? – Time management helps

Our quick-paced and stressful era makes it difficult for many people to get their body back in shape. However, sedentary activities combined with an incorrect nutrition take their toll, and that usually includes being overweight. Anybody who wants to reduce his weight should develop a special conscience for sport and must most certainly have a set time planning which includes regular training.

Efficient time planning is an important element, if running training is to be successful. Even before starting a running season, even a beginner can set himself realistic goals, and even make reservations for regional competitions. This makes it possible to set priorities which encourage a person to not sacrifice the important time for a running training.

Once a runner has achieved his goal, or even participated in a running competition, he will be more strongly motivated to increase his running success. But it is also possible to have phases which cause setbacks and initially leave the runner without motivation to continue practicing sport. Anybody will find a helpful support in the numerous running encounters, organized by several fitness studios and which don't force you to be a member.

If the motivation is at a low point, anybody can visualize the unbeatable benefits of a running training. Thus, running is not just important training for the heart and the circulatory system; it is also a type of sport that requires no expensive equipment. The sport can be carried out without problems at any time and everywhere and it offers the benefit, for overweight people, that it burns more calories than other types of sports. Beyond that, nowadays running is applied as an effective means to combat stress.

Combating the extra pounds – jogging as a fat burner and a panacea

Many people with fat pads who understood that a diet by itself won't cause a significant fat reduction can stimulate the burning of fat with regular running training.

It is proven that running you spend more calories than, for example, swimming or cycling. An endurance run at a low speed will burn more calories than intensive walking with full commitment of the body.

But it is not just body fat that disappears with regular training. People who suffer from sleeping disorders recover a relaxing sleep when they carry out regular training sessions.

Running as an effective means to reduce stress is a knowledge that is not precisely new. Many relaxing techniques don't have the effect caused by a running training in fresh air. What's more, this will increase the body's capabilities and strengthen its defenses.

Even slow running will promote health in the long term, since the heart and the circulatory system will get strengthened, and well-directed perseverance training will also strengthen the musculoskeletal system. Our sedentary society doesn't offer many chances to improve circulation or to strengthen the immune system.

Lose weight quickly and healthily by jogging

To be able to lose weight by jogging, the Calorie intake through food must be less than the daily use. A rule of thumb is that 1 Calorie is used per kilogram of body weight and kilometer run. Thus, if a man who weighs 70 kg (154.32 lbs) runs 10 km, he just uses up 700 Calories.

To use up the Calories of a 350 g (0.77 lbs) frozen pizza, you would have to jog 49-54 minutes, depending on the speed at which you run. 1 bottle (0.5 liters) of Pils requires 12-14 minutes of jogging, while a bar of milk chocolate requires 32-35 minutes.

If you want to lose weight by jogging, frequency is of the essence. You won't be successful by jogging once a week. Twice a week is enough to keep fit. It is convenient to run three times a week; after every run, there should be a free day for regeneration. Precisely when you are just starting it can be hard; in that case you should try to do Nordic walking between two running days. However, it will take at least two weeks before you get a visible success with respect to losing weight.

The food should be made up according to the 50-25-25 rule. That means that 50% of the food should consist of specific carbohydrates, and 25% each of healthy fats and protein.

Carbohydrates

The greatest energy suppliers are carbohydrates, which should be consumed at 6 grams (0.00086 lbs) per kg (2.205 lbs) of body weight. For a man who weighs 70 kg (154.32 lbs), this would be 420 g (0.93 lbs) per day. The carbohydrates are stored in the liver and muscles in form of glycogen. The energy thus saved is enough for 1.5 hours of endurance exercises. For untrained people, the storage capacity in carbohydrates is ca. 400 g 0.88 lbs). When the nutrition is optimized and there is regular training, the storage capacity can be increased to 600 (1.32lbs).

For the carbohydrates supply, you should give priority to whole grain products, cereal flakes, muesli, fruits and vegetables (preferably uncooked), whole grain noodles, potatoes and legumes.

The advantage of whole grain products is that the blood sugar level is kept constant, and therefore the productivity is also constant. They avoid a high insulin value; insulin inhibits the fat metabolism.

Carbohydrates with a high glycemic index, for example sweets, white flour products or glucose provide a high blood sugar level only for a short time; then it quickly goes down again, resulting in the strain of too little sugar.

In the evenings you should refrain from consuming carbohydrates, to lose weight faster.

Fats

Fats are also an energy supply. As a percentage, fat consumption is higher when running slowly, but in absolute terms it is lower.

In the case of fats, it is important to use mainly vegetal oils, which contain unsaturated or polyunsaturated fatty acids. Ideally olive oil, thistle oil, sunflower oil, or maize germ oil; but you should also pay attention to the amount.

Lean meat such as poultry or wild game meat as well as fish can be eaten. Wild game meat is especially good since it contains L-carnitine. L-carnitine has a special role for burning fats in combination with movement: it helps transport the fat into the energy-consuming cells. One recommendation is to consume 3 g (0.0066 lbs) of L-carnitine a day; the substance which is similar to amino-acids can be obtained from pharmacies or sport shops as capsule, powder or liquid, often as an additive in protein powder.

Fat can be additionally reduced by consuming lean cottage cheese, lean yoghurt, and by using lean varieties of sausage and cheese. A salad dressing can be made tasty with lean yoghurt, mustard and fresh herbs; or you can use sour cream instead of cream.

Protein

Proteins consist of amino-acids. The body can make some proteins itself; others must be taken in with food. The DGE (Deutsche Gesellschaft für Ernährung; German Nutrition Society) recommends a daily intake of 0.8 g (0.00177 lbs) per kg (2.205 lbs) of body weight as sufficient. High-performance athletes only require an additional 0.1 g (0,000014lbs) per kg (2.205 lbs) of body weight. Therefore it is not necessary to consume additional proteins, since the average protein intake is 1.2-1.4 grams 0.0026 lbs–0.0031 lbs) per kg (2.205 lbs) body weight.

It is convenient to combine protein intake from animal and vegetal products. That way, the body receives every essential amino-acid (i.e. amino-acids which the body can't produce itself).

Good combinations include potatoes and egg or cereals (for example muesli) with lean milk.

Minerals

The body loses minerals through sweat. Minerals that are especially important for the healthy functioning of the muscles are potassium and magnesium. Potassium is found in bananas, potatoes, milk and soya products, as well as dried fruits. Magnesium is contained in fruits and vegetables as well as whole grain products.

As a result of menstruation, women often suffer from a lack of iron. After consulting with a physician, this should be compensated, since iron is important for the body's oxygen supply.

Vitamins

Vitamins are very important for runners, especially vitamins C, E and B1. With a high-quality and varied nutrition, the vitamin requirements can be satisfied by food.

Vitamins are important for regulating the metabolism. They also strengthen the immune system and participate in cell building. They also have an antioxidant effect, that is, when the body is under stress free radicals are released which subject the body to an oxidative stress. This may cause aging processes or chronic diseases.

According to research, additional vitamin intake through food supplements doesn't improve sports performance.

Power bars and energy drinks

Experts generally recommend not to consume power bars. Power bars contain too much fat, usually trans-fatty acids, that is, industrially hardened plant fats which are responsible for an increased amount of LDL-cholesterol in the blood. LDL-cholesterol has negative effects for diseases such as arteriosclerosis and heart attacks.

Energy drinks, lemonades, and cola drinks are not recommended due to their high sugar contents. Drinking however is important, since you sweat while doing sports, and this loss of liquid must be compensated. Before and during sports, the body should be supplied by isotonic drinks. Isotonic means that the drink has the same amount of dissolved substances as the blood. Fruit juice spritzers are ideal, especially the apple spritzer in the ratio 1:1 or 1:2 juice to mineral water. The spritzer, however, should have no sugar. Also, please don't use light products, or products that contain aspartame or another sugar replacement.

Weight control

It should be noted that muscle mass is heavier than fat. Therefore it is possible for weight to remain constant, even if fat is burned. You get information about the actual fat loss with a fat scale that shows the body's fat percentage.

To control the body weight, it is convenient to weigh yourself every day in the morning after going to the bathroom, without clothing. That way you have uniform conditions, but these will also inform you when you have "sinned".

Don't eat late at night

At night, ca. 3 hours before going to bed, you shouldn't eat anything. If you really can't do without the bad habit of eating chips, sweets or similar things when watching television, you should at least eat fruits or lean, protein-rich chicken breast or turkey, with lemon juice and without garnishes.

Final comments

Running is an ideal sport to train your entire musculoskeletal system. Many muscle groups are used when running. As a result, the metabolism is increased within a short time, achieving a fat-reducing effect.

A great side effect when running are the bodily and mental fruits that you can get: you will lose weight precisely in the problem areas, get more capable of withstanding stress, have more moments of happiness, more stress resistance and won't get sick as easily, since the immune system is strengthened tremendously. In general you'll get more self-confident and capable.

You'll be more content and balanced, and all this without investing a lot of money.

Now I wish you a lot of fun during your running training.